Nurse's Toolbox

A Comprehensive Guide to Clinical Nursing Skills

Dr. Kai Finch-Hatton
Senior Nurse Educator, Royal Melbourne Hospital, Australia.

Lecture note series,
June, 2024.

©2024.Dr. Kai Finch-Hatton

Reproduction, distribution, or transmission of any part of this publication, in any form or by any means, whether electronic, mechanical, photocopying, recording, or otherwise is prohibited without the publisher's prior written consent. Exceptions are granted for brief quotations used in critical reviews or other noncommercial purposes permitted by copyright law.

Foreword

Nursing stands at the forefront of healthcare delivery systems, where a multitude of strategies, from health promotion to disease prevention, curative interventions, and rehabilitative measures are employed. The clinical prowess of nurses holds paramount importance, not only in delivering comprehensive care but also in enhancing clinical proficiency. This preface serves to introduce a lecture note series aimed at equipping nurses with fundamental clinical nursing skills, fostering their ability to fulfill their responsibilities effectively.

The lecture note series is structured into two parts: Part I focuses on essential clinical skills, while Part II delves into advanced clinical skills and fundamental concepts related to these skills. It is widely acknowledged that basic clinical nursing skills form the cornerstone of nursing practice. These skills are indispensable for nurses providing healthcare across various settings, including hospitals, health centers, health posts, and within communities, where home-based care for chronically ill patients is paramount. Furthermore, it is anticipated that primary and middle-level health professional training institutions will utilize these lecture notes to effectively hone their students' professional skills.

Organized in a logical progression, the lecture notes enable students to grasp concepts from the simplest to the most complex. Also incorporated in this note are important abbreviations and key terminologies to facilitate the teaching-learning process. Additionally, clear learning objectives are outlined to guide students towards the desired outcomes. A glossary is provided at the end to elucidate terminologies introduced as learning stimuli at the onset of each section, alongside the corresponding learning objectives. Scientific explanations for procedures are offered wherever possible, supplemented by relevant study questions to deepen students' comprehension of the subject matter. Furthermore, to promote a systematic approach to nursing care delivery, the nursing process is delineated for most procedures.

ACKNOWLEDGEMENT

I am profoundly grateful to Dr. Jordan Bessell-Browne, MD, PhD, Chief of Cardiology, Royal Melbourne Hospital, Australia, for his invaluable guidance and support throughout the creation of this book, Nurse's Toolbox:A Comprehensive Guide to Clinical Nursing Skills. His extensive expertise and unwavering dedication to advancing clinical education have been a tremendous inspiration.

Dr. Bessell-Browne's insights and feedback have been instrumental in shaping the content and ensuring its relevance and accuracy. His commitment to excellence in patient care and medical education is reflected in every page of this book. I am deeply honored to have had the opportunity to work with such a distinguished and compassionate professional.

Thank you, Dr. Bessell-Browne's for your mentorship, encouragement, and unwavering belief in the importance of nurturing the next generation of nursing professionals. This book would not have been possible without your remarkable contributions.

Dr. Kai Finch-Hatton
Senior Nurse Educator
Royal Melbourne Hospital

CONTENT

Forward

Acknowledgement

Introduction to Nursing Education and Practice
- Definition
- Learning Objectives

Nursing Through History
- Historical Background
- Traditional Perceptions
- The Nurse as Mother
- The Nurse as God's Worker
- The Renaissance Image
- The Nurse as Attendant
- The Emergence of Modern Nursing

Nursing Process and Critical Thinking

- Purpose and Steps of the Nursing Process
- Assessment
- Diagnosis
- Planning
- Implementation
- Evaluation
- Establishing Expected Outcomes
- Selecting Nursing Interventions
- Critical Thinking in Nursing

Safety in Health Care Facilities and Infection Control
- Learning Objectives
- Universal Precautions
- Factors Predisposing to Infection
- Specimen Collection Techniques

Patient Care Skills
- Bed Making
- Cleansing Bath
- Care for Perineum
- Hair Care
- Pediculosis Treatment
- Feeding a Helpless Patient

- Evening Care

Cold and Heat Therapy
- Learning Objectives
- Patient Care for Fever
- Local Application of Cold and Heat

Body Mechanics and Mobility
- Learning Objectives
- Basic Principles of Body Mechanics
- Positioning the Client
- Moving and Positioning Clients
- Joint Mobility and Range of Motion
- Controlling Postural Hypotension
- Crutch Walking

Nutrition and Metabolism
- Fluid, Electrolyte, and Acid-Base Balance
- Nutrition Principles

Medication Administration
- Learning Objectives
- Drug Metabolism
- Drug Administration

- Different Routes of Administration

Wound Care
- Learning Objectives
- Wound Classification
- Wound Healing
- Dressing Techniques
- Wound Irrigation
- Suturing and Stitch Removal

Perioperative Nursing Care (Pre & Postoperative Nursing Care)
- Learning Objectives
- Preoperative Preparation
- Postoperative Measures
- Specific Post-operative Care

End-of-Life Care and Postmortem Care
- Learning Objectives
- Care of the Dying
- Nursing Process Assessment
- Care After Death

Glossary

Abbreviations & Symbols

ABG - Arterial Blood Gas
Ab - Antibody
ABCDE: exposure, examination, breathing, circulation, and disability
ABCDE: exposure, examination, breathing, circulation, and disability

A.C. - Before meal (ante cibum)
ACTH - Adreno trophic hormone
AD. - As desired
ADL - Activities of daily living
AIDS - Acquired immunodeficiency syndrome
AI - Adequate intake
AM. - Morning
AMALG - Amalgam filling
AMA - Against medical advice
A and P - Auscultation and percussion
APC - Aspirin, Phenacetin & caffeine
AP - Apical pulse or antero-posterior
AQ - Aqueous

A-R - Apical radial pulse
AROM - Active range of motion; artificial rupture of membrane
Ax - Axillary
BID - Twice a day (bis in die)
B.M - Bowel movement
B.M.R. - Basal metabolic rate
B.P - Blood pressure
BPM - Beat per minute
B.R.P. - Bathroom privilege
BUN - Blood urea nitrogen
oC - Centigrade
CBC - Complete blood count
CC - Cubic centimeter
C.N. S. - Central nervous system
Co2 - Carbon dioxide
C.S. F. - Cerebro-spinal fluid
CXR - Chest X-ray
D and C - Dilatation and Curettage
D/NS - Dextrose in normal saline
DPT - Diphtheria, pertussis, tetanus
D/W - Dextrose in water
Dx - Diagnosis
EEG - Electroencephalogram

E.E.N.T. - Eye, ear, nose, throat
ECG - Electrocardiogram
oF - Fahrenheit
F.B.S. - Fasting blood sugar
F.H.B. - Fetal heartbeat
Gastrointestinal
G or Gm - Gram
gr. - Grain
gt. - Drop (gutte)
gtt. - Drops
G.U. - Genitourinary
GYN. - Gynecology
HCL - Hydrochloric acid
Hb - Hemoglobin
HS - At bed-time (hours of sleep)
H2o - Water
I.V. - Intravenous
I.V.P - Intravenous pyelogram
KI. - Potassium iodide
L. P - Lumbar puncture
NaCl - Sodium Chloride
NOCTE - At night
NPO: Nothing via OS (nothing orally) NPO: Nothing via OS (nothing orally)

O.P.D. - OutPatient Department
O.R. - Operating room
PM - Afternoon
PRN - As needed, when necessary
Pt. - Patient
Q. - Every
Q.D. - Every Day
Q.H. - Every Hour
Q.I.D. - Four times a day
Q.N. - Every night
Q.O.D. - Every other day
RBC stands for red blood cell or red blood count.
Rh. - Rhesus factor
Rx - Prescription, take
Sol. - Solution
SOS - If necessary
STAT - Immediately -at once
S.C - Subcutaneous
T. I.D - Three times a day
T.P.R. - Temperature, pulse, respiration
Tsp - Teaspoon, tablespoon
U.R. - Upper right

WBC - White blood cells
Wt. - Weight
U.R.Q. - Upper right quadrant
U.L.Q. - Upper lower quadrant
UTI - Urinary tract Infection

Introduction to Nursing Education and Practice

Learning Objectives:
Upon completing this unit, learners will be able to:
- Define nursing according to modern standards
- Provide an overview of nursing's historical evolution globally
- Recognize the significant contributions of individuals in the field of nursing
- Explain the nursing process
- Understand critical thinking as a tool for delivering high-quality care

Nursing Through History

Definition

According to the American Nurses Association (1980), nursing includes the diagnosis and treatment of human reactions to current or impending health crises.

It involves aiding individuals, whether healthy or sick, in activities contributing to health or recovery, promoting independence as swiftly as possible.

Nursing is a blend of art and science, involving collaboration with individuals, families, and communities to enhance physical, mental, and spiritual well-being. It serves as a dynamic, therapeutic, and educational process, addressing the health needs of society, particularly its most vulnerable members.

Historical Background of Nursing

Nursing boasts a history as ancient as humanity itself. Throughout history, humans have grappled with the challenge of maintaining health and caring for the sick and dependent. Those proficient in this domain stood out, sometimes passing their skills to others. Uprichard (1973) categorized nursing's early history using three archetypes: the folk image, the religious image, and the renaissance image.

The Traditional Perception of Nursing: The Nurse as Mother

The early development of nursing, scantily documented, necessitates speculation based on knowledge of ancient civilizations. Nurses typically belonged to families or communities, demonstrating exceptional care skills. Nursing was perceived as an extension of maternal roles, prevalent in early historical records and persisting in primitive cultures.

The Nurse as God's Worker: A Religious Perspective on Nursing

In religious contexts, nursing was linked to service. Biblical references, like Phoebe, the first deaconess, highlight care for the sick, widows, and orphans. Various religious orders, such as monks and nuns, continued this tradition, establishing hospitals and caring for the ill. Unfortunately, during the Middle Ages, knowledge of hygiene and sanitation waned, stagnating healthcare practices.

Throughout the Middle Ages and into the Reformation era, religious institutions predominantly operated hospitals and provided nursing care across Europe. However, with the onset of the Reformation and the emergence of Protestant religious factions, the dynamics of these institutions underwent significant changes. Women began joining religious orders for finite periods rather than committing to lifelong service, echoing the early church's concept of deaconesses. Pastor Theodor Fleidner of Kaiserswerth, Germany, established a church order of deaconesses known as the Sisters of Mercy of the Church of England. Similarly, another order founded St. John's House, an Anglican Hospital in London. While Protestant nursing groups were predominantly composed of women, only one nursing order comprised men, namely the Brothers Hospitalers of St. John, which remained within the Catholic Church. In the Muslim faith, a similar tradition of serving others in the name of God exists. Rofiada al Islamiah, one of the wives of Muhammad, is revered as the mother of nursing in the Middle Eastern Muslim countries for her compassionate care of the sick and injured (Meleis, 1985).

The Renaissance Image of Nursing

The Nurse as Attendant

During the Renaissance, there was a decline in monastic orders and a surge in individualism and materialism. This period marked a stark departure from the earlier perception of the selfless nurse, prevalent in the early Christian era and the Middle Ages. The responsibility of caring for the sick was often delegated to servants or individuals with limited means of support. Hospitals of this era were marred by disease and death, with those working in them often viewed as corrupt and unsavory.

The Emergence of Modern Nursing

For centuries, the three archetypes of nursing coexisted. However, in the 19th century, a single individual revolutionized the field: Florence Nightingale. Despite being born into privilege and Victorian English Society, Nightingale held steadfast to Christian ideals and eschewed a life of luxury. She believed her true calling lay in tending to the sick. Recognizing that optimal care required education, Nightingale embarked on personal study and research into sanitation and health, even studying under Pastor Fleidner of 33, who reorganized care for the sick at a hospital for 'Gentlewomen in Distressed Circumstances.'

Nightingale's success led Britain's secretary of war to enlist her for a more daunting task: reforming healthcare in the Crimean War. Arriving at the frontlines, Nightingale was appalled by the deplorable conditions in military hospitals. Taking control of supplies, funds, and personnel, she and her team reduced the death rate among wounded soldiers from over 50% to less than 3%. Her efforts revolutionized the British military's approach to healthcare.

In 1860, Nightingale established a nursing school, serving as the model for nursing education in England. Emphasizing a trained matron's authority, a comprehensive theoretical and practical curriculum, and moral and spiritual training overseen by "sisters," Nightingale set rigorous educational standards. Her school prepared nurses for various roles, including hospital care and public health. Nightingale's advocacy for nurses' roles and lifelong education cemented nursing as a respected profession.

Before modern nursing, medical practice was intertwined with religious rituals. Nomadic tribe women and caregiving mothers tended to the young, old, and sick, laying the foundation for nursing practices. As society evolved through religious, economic, and industrial changes, nursing also expanded, culminating in modern nursing during Florence Nightingale's era. Her legacy continues to shape nursing globally.

NURSING PROCESS AND CRITICAL THINKING

Definition: The Nursing Process serves as a structured approach to organizing and delivering care, representing a methodical intellectual endeavor in nursing practice. It encompasses systematic problem-solving aimed at addressing client needs, comprising planned steps and actions to meet those needs and resolve associated issues (Sorensen and Luckman, 1986).

Purpose of Nursing Process:

To identify clients' healthcare needs
To formulate nursing care plans tailored to meet those needs
To execute nursing interventions designed to address the identified needs
To provide individualized care

Steps of the Nursing Process:

Assessment: This step involves the systematic collection of data to ascertain the patient's health status and identify actual or potential health problems. The primary sources of information include the client and family, supplemented by healthcare professionals, previous records, and significant others. Data collected can be objective (measurable and observable) or subjective (client's opinions and feelings).

Methods of data collection include observation, health interviews, and physical examination.

Diagnosis: This step entails identifying nursing and collaborative diagnoses, with nursing diagnoses referring to actual or potential health problems manageable through independent nursing interventions.

The purposes of nursing diagnosis include setting priorities, guiding interventions, facilitating communication, forming the basis for quality assurance, aiding evaluation, and informing staffing decisions.

Diagnostic Statement: A diagnostic statement typically consists of the problem, etiology, and signs and symptoms. The problem describes the health issue succinctly using NANDA-approved nursing diagnostic labels, while etiology identifies its cause, and signs and symptoms summarize relevant data.

Writing the Diagnostic Statement: The statement links the problem and etiology with "related to" and the problem, signs and symptoms with "as evidenced by."

Collaborative Problems: These involve physiologic complications monitored by nurses to detect changes in status, managed through physician-prescribed and nursing-prescribed interventions.

Planning: This step involves goal development and care plan formulation to aid the patient in resolving diagnosed problems. Prioritization is crucial, with survival needs taking precedence.

Establishing Expected Outcomes

An expected outcome, also termed as a goal or objective, refers to a measurable client behavior indicating the achievement of expected benefits from nursing care. Such outcomes possess the following characteristics:

Client-oriented
Specific
Reasonable
Measurable

Selecting Nursing Interventions

Nursing interventions, alternatively known as nursing orders or actions, encompass activities likely to yield desired outcomes, whether short-term or long-term. Examples of nursing interventions include:

Offering fluids frequently
Repositioning regularly
Teaching deep breathing exercises
Monitoring vital signs
Administering oxygen, among others

Implementation involves the actualization of the care plan through nursing interventions, followed by evaluation to ascertain the patient's responses and goal achievement.

Critical Thinking

Critical thinking denotes an intellectually disciplined process of actively and skillfully conceptualizing, applying, analyzing, synthesizing, and evaluating information gathered from observation, experience, reflection, reasoning, or communication, guiding belief and action. It encompasses problem-solving and decision-making, involving competencies such as diagnostic reasoning, clinical inferences, and clinical decision-making, which are integral to nursing practice. Critical thinking aids in examining ideas, beliefs, principles, assumptions, conclusions, statements, and inferences before drawing conclusions and making decisions.

Safety in Health Care Facilities and Infection Control

Learning Objectives:

Describe infection prevention in healthcare settings
List the chain of infection
Differentiate between medical asepsis and surgical asepsis
Discuss the purpose, use, and components of standard precautions
Maintain both medical and surgical asepsis
Describe how to set up a client's room for isolation, including appropriate barrier techniques
Explain the appropriate ways to adhere to specific droplet, contact, and airborne safety measures.

The Chain of Infection consists of six interrelated links:

1. Etiologic agent, referring to the microorganism causing the infection.
2. Reservoir, the natural habitat where the organism resides.
3. Portal of exit from the reservoir.
4. Method of transmission.
5. Portal of entry into the host.
6. Susceptibility of the host.

Factors Predisposing to Infection

Various circumstances and invasive procedures increase the susceptibility of patients to infections by compromising the integrity of the skin or creating conditions conducive to the development of infection. Common predisposing factors include surgical incisions, changes in the body's antibacterial defense mechanisms, or underlying illnesses.

Hospital-Acquired Infections

Nosocomial infections are those acquired by patients during their stay in a medical facility, infections that were neither present nor in the incubation stage upon admission.

Standard Precautions

Standard precautions, also known as universal precautions, were implemented in response to the HIV epidemic. These precautions involved the practice of blood and body fluid safety measures with all patients, irrespective of their infectious status.

In 1987, body substance isolation (BSI) was introduced, aiming to contain all moist and potentially infectious bodily substances (such as blood, urine, feces, sputum, saliva, wound drainage, and other bodily
fluids), generally with the use of gloves, from all patients, irrespective of their state of infection.

Standard precautions combine the key aspects of universal precautions (blood and body fluid precautions) and body substance isolation into a unified set of precautions to be applied to all patients regardless of their supposed infection status or diagnosis, in healthcare settings.

These precautions encompass blood, all body fluids, secretions, excretions (regardless of the presence of visible blood), non-intact skin, and mucous membranes.

Essential Principles: Certain fundamental practices should be applied to all patients, including hand hygiene, glove use, proper patient placement within the healthcare setting to prevent microbial spread, and appropriate utilization of isolation equipment to prevent microbial transmission to healthcare workers and other patients.

Specimen Collection:

Specimen collection involves gathering various samples, including stool, urine, blood, and other bodily fluids or tissues, from patients for diagnostic or therapeutic purposes. These samples are collected in clinical settings, either in outpatient departments (OPDs) or inpatient units, to aid in diagnosis and treatment.

General Considerations for Specimen Collection:

1. Wear gloves to protect against contact with body fluids.
2. Obtain a request for specimen collection, identifying the type of specimen and the patient.
3. Provide adequate explanation to the patient regarding the purpose and method of collection.
4. Organize necessary materials and label specimen containers accurately.
5. Promptly send specimens to the laboratory to prevent temperature or time-related alterations.

Collecting Stool Specimens:
Purpose:

- For laboratory diagnosis, including microscopic examination and culture and sensitivity tests.

Equipment Required:

- Clean bedpan or commode
- Wooden spatula or applicator
- Specimen container
- Tissue paper
- Disposable gloves (for patients confined to bed)
- Bed protecting materials
- Screen

Procedure:

- Provide instructions to ambulatory patients or assist bed-confined patients.
- Make sure the patient is comfortable and has privacy.
- Collect stool samples into the designated container using a spatula or applicator.

- Handle and label the specimen correctly and promptly send it to the laboratory.
- Dispose of the bedpan's contents and clean equipment appropriately.

Documentation and Reporting:
Record relevant data, including specimen type, amount, time, and date of collection, and report any abnormalities.

Collecting Urine Specimens:

Types of Urine Specimen Collection:
- Clean voided urine specimen
- Sterile urine specimen
- Timed urine specimen (short or long period)

Purpose:

- For diagnostic purposes, including routine laboratory analysis and culture and sensitivity tests.

Equipment Required:

- Disposable gloves
- Specimen container
- Laboratory requisition form
- Water and soap or antiseptic solutions (for cleaning)
- Urine receptacles (for bed-confined patients)
- Bed protecting materials
- Screen (if needed)

Procedure:

- Provide instructions and assist patients as necessary.
- Collect midstream urine into the specimen container, avoiding contamination.
- Handle and label the container correctly and promptly send it to the laboratory.
- Dispose of receptacle contents properly and clean equipment.
- Document pertinent data, including specimen details and patient experience.

These procedures ensure accurate specimen collection and facilitate proper diagnosis and treatment for patients.

Collecting a Sterile Urine Specimen:
A sterile urine specimen is obtained using a catheter with aseptic techniques. Detailed instructions for this procedure are provided in the catheterization section.

Collecting a Timed Urine Specimen:
Purpose:

- For specific renal function tests and urine composition assessments, such as measuring hormone levels (e.g., adrenocorticosteroid hormone), creatinine clearance, or protein quantitation.

Equipment Required:

- Urine specimen collection materials provided by the laboratory and stored in the patient's bathroom.

- Record format for documenting the start and end times, date, and urine volume collected during each voiding period.

Procedure:
Patient Preparation:

- Explain the purpose of the test to the patient and provide instructions on what to do with the urine.
- Place alert signs about specimen collection in the patient's room or bathroom.

Label the specimen container with the date, time of each voiding, and patient identification.
Containers may be sequentially numbered (e.g., 1st, 2nd, 3rd) for 24-hour urine collection.

Collecting Urine:

- Typically starts in the morning.
- Instruct the patient to void before beginning the timed collection (discard this urine).

- Collect all urine voided during the specified period (e.g., the next 24 hours) in the container.
- At the end of the collection period, have the patient void one final specimen, which is added to the collected urine.
- Ensure the urine is free of feces.

Collecting Sputum Specimen:

Sputum, distinct from saliva, is the mucus secretion from the lungs, bronchi, and trachea. The optimal time for collection is in the morning upon waking, when accumulated overnight. If the patient cannot cough out sputum, the nurse may aspirate pharyngeal secretions using suction.

Purpose:

- Sputum specimens are typically collected for culture and sensitivity tests, cytological examination, acid-fast bacillus (AFB) tests, and therapy effectiveness assessment.

Equipment Required:

- Disposable gloves
- Specimen container
- Laboratory requisition form
- Mouth care (wash) tray

Procedure:

Patient Preparation:
- Educate the patient on distinguishing between sputum and saliva and how to cough deeply to raise sputum.
- Position the patient upright, utilize splinting or postural drainage as needed.
- Provide oral care to minimize mouth microorganism contamination.

Obtaining Sputum Specimen:

- Don gloves to prevent contact, especially in cases of hemoptysis (blood in sputum).
- Instruct the patient to cough deeply to produce sputum.

- Collect approximately 15-30 ml of sputum in the specimen container.
- Ensure the container's outer surface remains uncontaminated; clean if necessary.
- Seal the container securely.

Comfort the patient and provide post-collection oral care to eliminate any unpleasant taste.

Handle and label the specimen container appropriately and promptly send it to the laboratory. Ensure proper care of used equipment.

Document the sputum's amount, color, consistency (thick, watery, tenacious), and presence of blood.

General Rules for Charting:

Spelling:
Ensure accurate spelling in all entries.

Accuracy:

Maintain precise and truthful records in every aspect.

Completeness:
Avoid omitting any necessary information and refrain from including unnecessary words or statements.

Exactness:
Only use words with which you are confident and certain.

Objective Information:
Record observable details rather than subjective interpretations (e.g., avoid stating conditions better).

Legibility:
Write or print clearly and distinctly, making entries easily readable.

Neatness:
Present charts without wrinkles, ensuring proper placement of items.

Abbreviations:
Use abbreviations sparingly and consistently, listing them at the end of each entry.

Composition/Arrangement:
Carefully organize chart entries, avoiding chemical formulas and ensuring clear, complete sentences without repetition.

Avoid Overwriting:
Prevent excessive crossing out or rewriting in chart entries.

Spacing:
Do not leave empty spaces between entries.

Time of Charting:
Specify the exact time and date of each entry.

Ink Color:
Use black or blue ink for standard entries, reserving red for special cases such as transfusions or surgical days.

Charting Procedures:

All orders must be written and signed, with verbal or telephone orders documented only in emergencies and then transcribed onto the order sheet and signed during the next visit.

Orders of Assembling Patient Charts:
1. History sheet
2. Personal and social data
3. Order sheet
4. Doctor's progress notes
5. Nurses' notes
6. Vital sign sheet (graphics)
7. Intake and output recording sheet
8. Laboratory and other diagnostic reports

Patient or family access to charts is restricted unless permitted by the patient.

Intake and Output:
- Intake includes all fluids taken orally, through NG tubes, or intravenously.

- Output comprises all fluids excreted through the mouth, urethra, or other routes, including GI losses like diarrhea or vomiting.

Purpose of Intake and Output Recording:
- Replacing fluid losses
- Providing maintenance requirements
- Checking for fluid retention

Fluid Balance Sheet:
Compare intake and output over a 24-hour period, recording a positive balance if intake exceeds output and a negative balance if output exceeds intake.

Patient Care Skills

Bed Making:

Creating a Postoperative Bed

Ensure the entire bed has clean linen. Start by making the bottom of the bed as usual. It is usually necessary to place a draw sheet under the client's hips and another under their head when using a postoperative bed. Depending on the case, top linens may be folded at the foot of the bed or a full postoperative bed may be made.

To accomplish this, place the top linens over the foundation without tucking them in. Fold down the top similar to an occupied bed, then fold the bottom of the linens up to align with the mattress's bottom. Do not tuck in the linens. Fanfold the top linens to the side opposite the client's stretcher or to the foot of the bed, leaving a tab for easy grabbing.

Have at least two pillows available but refrain from placing them on the bed unless deemed safe by the physician or charge nurse. Ensure furniture is out of the way, and keep the call light accessible on the bedside stand until the client is in bed. The call light cord should be positioned to facilitate the client's transfer to bed. Before determining the necessary special equipment, ascertain the surgical procedure the client underwent. Additionally, make tissues, an emesis basin, a blood pressure cuff and stethoscope, a "frequent vital signs" flow sheet, an intake and output record, and an IV stand available according to the client's specific needs. Notify the charge nurse upon completing the postoperative bed and assembling the required equipment.

Procedures for other beds, such as cardiac beds, are similar, with additional considerations like including an overbed table and extra pillows for cardiac patients and utilizing a hardboard under the mattress for fracture beds.

Cleansing Bath:

Providing a cleansing bath serves primarily for hygiene purposes and encompasses various types:

Complete Bed Bath: In this method, the nurse washes the entire body of a dependent patient while they remain in bed.

Self-Help Bed Bath: This approach allows bed-confined clients to bathe themselves, with assistance from the nurse for areas like the back and possibly the face.

Partial Bath (Abbreviated Bath): Only specific parts of the client's body that may cause discomfort or odor if neglected are washed, such as the face, hands, axilla, perineum, and back (the nurse can aid in washing the back), while omitting the arms, chest, and abdomen.

Tub Bath: This method is preferable to bed baths as it facilitates easier washing and rinsing in a tub, also commonly used for therapeutic purposes.

Shower: Ambulatory clients can often utilize a shower for bathing.

The water temperature should be comfortably warm for the client, typically ranging from 43-46°C (110-115°F). However, individual sensitivity to heat varies, so it's essential to consider the client's comfort level.

Before bathing a patient, ascertain the type of bath required, the level of assistance needed, any other ongoing care the client is receiving to prevent undue fatigue, and the necessary bed linen.

It's crucial to wear gloves when bathing a client with an infection, especially in the presence of body fluids or open lesions.

Principles:

Close doors and windows to prevent heat loss via convection.

Ensure privacy for the client's comfort and dignity.

Encourage the client to avoid before the bath for convenience.

Position the bed at a height that reduces strain on the nurse's back.

Assist the client in moving closer to facilitate access during bathing.

Use a bath mitt made from a washcloth to retain water and heat better.

To stop the spread of germs and the entry of secretions into the nasolacrimal duct, clean the eyes from the inner to the outer canthus using different washcloth corners.

Apply firm strokes from distal to proximal parts of the extremities to enhance venous blood return.

Purpose:

The cleansing bath aims to remove transient moisture, body secretions, and dead skin cells, stimulate circulation, promote relaxation and cleanliness, prevent or eliminate unpleasant body odors, provide an opportunity for nursing assessment, and prevent pressure sores.

Two categories of baths are typically administered to clients: cleansing and therapeutic.

Technique for Back Massage:

Massage the back by stroking towards the neckline using long, firm, and smooth strokes.

Pause at the neckline and use your fingers to massage the sides of the neck gently.

With a kneading motion, massage outwards along the shoulders, continuing this motion down each side of the trunk with both hands until you return to the sacral area.

Place your hands side by side with palms down and rub in figure-eight patterns over the buttocks and sacral area.

Adjust the pressure according to the client's preference, applying light pressure for smoothing and heavier pressure for stimulation.

Continue with the kneading motion, moving up the sides around the vertebrae through the interscapular space towards the shoulders.

Ask the client if there are any specific areas they would like to focus on.

Finish the back rub with long, firm strokes up and down the back, from shoulder to sacrum and back to shoulder.

Comfort the client and use a towel to mop any excess oil or lotion from their back. If the skin is moist, apply powder or alcohol to further dry it.

Assist the client in dressing, replace the top cover, and reposition them comfortably.

Leave the client in a comfortable position.

Ensure proper care of all equipment used during the massage.

Document the procedure, including observations and the client's reactions. Report any abnormal findings on the skin, such as signs of pressure sores, to the nurse or physician in charge.

Three Types of Massage Strokes:

Effleurage: Involves stroking the body with light, circular friction and firm, straight strokes, which can have a relaxing sedative effect.

Petrissage: Includes kneading and making large, quick pinches of the skin, tissue, and muscle, stimulating if done quickly with firm pressure.

Assessment and Duration:

Assess for signs of relaxation or decreased pain, including relaxed breathing, decreased muscle tension, drowsiness, and a peaceful effect.

The duration of a massage typically ranges from 5 to 20 minutes, ensuring to avoid direct pressure over bony prominences to prevent discomfort.

Frequent repositioning is preferable to back massage to avoid potential subcutaneous tissue degeneration, especially in elderly clients.

Care for Female Perineum:

For convenient cleansing of the vulva and perineum, a woman can use a bedpan.

Secretions typically accumulate on the inner surface of the labia.

Gently retract the labia using one hand while using a separate section of a washcloth for each wipe, moving in a downward motion from the urethra to the back perineum. Then proceed to clean the rectal area.

Note: Following genital or rectal surgery, sterile supplies may be necessary for cleaning the operative site, such as sterile cotton balls. Antiseptic solutions may be applied to the perineum by squirting them from a squeeze bottle.

Male Perineum:

The penis contains pathways for urination and ejaculation through the urethral orifice (meatus), with the glans covered by a skin flap known as the foreskin or prepuce. The urethral orifice is centrally located and opens at the tip.

The shaft of the penis comprises erectile tissue bound by dense fibrous tissue of the foreskin.

To prevent embarrassment or discomfort, hold the shaft of the penis firmly with one hand while using the other hand to hold the washcloth. Clean the penis in a circular motion from the center to the periphery, using a separate section of the washcloth.

Position: For cleansing the perineal part, the patient can lie in bed with knees flexed, while side-lying is suitable for cleaning the perineal area. Always stroke from front to back to wash from clean to dirty' parts, as the urethral orifice is the cleanest area and the anal orifice is the dirtiest.

Hair Care:

Hair care is typically conducted after bathing and as a daily hygiene practice. It includes combing, washing/shampooing, and treatment for pediculosis.

Combing/Brushing of Hair:

Patients should comb or brush their hair daily to stimulate blood circulation to the scalp, distribute hair oils evenly, and promote a healthy sheen. This activity can increase the patient's sense of well-being.

Equipment needed includes a large-toothed comb, hand mirror, towel, and lubricant/oils if necessary.

Procedure:

Prepare the patient by positioning them comfortably, either sitting, semi-Fowler's, or lying flat if they are unable to sit. Place a towel over the patient's shoulder or pillow.

Remove any pins or ribbons from the hair. Divide the hair and comb each section from the ends towards the scalp to remove tangles. Continue until all hair is combed, arranging it neatly according to the patient's preference.

Comfort the patient, remove the towel, and ensure they are in a comfortable position.

Care for equipment and document the procedure.

Shampooing/Washing the Hair:

The purpose of shampooing/washing the hair is to stimulate blood circulation to the scalp, clean the hair for a sense of well-being, and treat hair disorders like dandruff.

Equipment needed includes a comb, brush, shampoo/soap, shampoo basin, plastic sheet, wash towels, cotton balls, water basin, and lubricants/oil if required.

Procedure:

Prepare the patient by assisting them to move to one side of the bed. Remove any hair accessories and brush/comb the hair to remove tangles.

Arrange the equipment by placing a plastic sheet under the patient's head and shoulder, tucking towels under the shoulder and neck, and positioning the shampoo basin under the patient's head with one end extending to a receptacle for used water.

Protect the patient's eyes and ears with damp washcloths and cotton balls.

Wet the hair thoroughly, apply shampoo/soap, and massage the scalp using fingertips. Rinse the hair with plain water, remove the washcloths and cotton balls, and dry the hair with a towel or hair dryer if available.

Ensure patient comfort, remove the plastic sheet and shampoo basin, assist the patient in grooming, and document the procedure.

Pediculosis Treatment:

Pediculosis refers to an infestation with lice and requires treatment to prevent the transmission of diseases and provide comfort to the patient.

Equipment needed includes Lindane or 1% permethrin cream rinse, clean linen, fine-tooth "nit" comb, disinfectant for the comb, clean gloves, and a towel.

Lice are small, grayish-white parasitic insects found on the scalp (pediculosis capitis), pubic hair (pediculosis pubis), and clothing (pediculosis).

Treatment options include DDT, kerosene oil, oil of sassafras, and Gammaxene. These treatments should be applied according to guidelines to effectively kill adult lice and nits.

Feeding a Helpless Patient:

Feeding a patient who is unable to feed themselves requires knowledge, sensitivity, and skill to ensure they receive adequate nutrition and promote their well-being.

Early morning, late morning, afternoon, and evening care are provided to clients at different times of the day to assist with hygiene and comfort needs. These routines include tasks such as providing a urinal or bedpan, bathing, oral care, and grooming.

Evening Care:

Evening care is administered to patients before they settle in for the night.

Tasks involved include:
Addressing elimination needs
Hand washing
Administering oral care
Providing back massage if necessary

Study Questions:
1. Define the objectives of bed bath, oral care, and perineal care.
2. Explain the concept of therapeutic bathing.
3. Enumerate the three categories of massage strokes utilized in back care.
4. Identify the suitable position for administering perineal care in both genders.

Cold and Heat Therapy

Learning Objectives:
By the end of this section, learners will be proficient in:
- Articulating the rationale behind applying heat and cold to the body.
- Detailing specific precautions when administering heat or cold therapy.
- Demonstrating the procedure for leg soaks and sitz baths.

Key Terminology:
- Hypothermia blanket
- Sitz bath
- Tepid sponge bath

Patient Care for Fever:
This encompasses gently sponging the skin with alcohol or cool water to reduce body temperature.
Solution: Tepid (lukewarm) water.

Alcohol Solution:

Mix one part of alcohol with three parts of lukewarm water and remove the patient's gown. Take the patient's temperature, then sponge the body using a washcloth alternately, spending 2-3 minutes on each part, changing the washcloth. Heat loss occurs via conduction or vaporization. Monitor the pulse frequently and report any changes.

Localized Application of Heat and Cold:

Both heat and cold are applied to the body for localized and systemic effects.

Purpose of Heat Application:
- Alleviate pain and muscle spasms by relaxing muscles.
- Increase blood flow to the area.
- Reduce swelling to facilitate wound healing.
- Alleviate inflammation and congestion.

Heat:

- Enhances the action of phagocytic cells, aiding in the removal of foreign material.
- Facilitates the elimination of waste products from metabolic processes.
- Provides comfort and alleviates chilling.

Dry Heat:
Applied locally for heat conduction, typically using a hot water bottle.

Moist Heat:
Administered through conduction, commonly via compression or sitz baths.

Purpose of Cold Application:
- Reduce pain by decreasing prostaglandins, which sensitize pain receptors.
- Diminish swelling and inflammation by constricting blood vessels.
- Lower elevated body temperature during fever episodes.

Cold can be applied in both moist (cold compress) and dry forms (ice pack).

Systemic effects:
Extensive cold application can elevate blood pressure, while hot applications can lower it due to excessive peripheral vasodilation.

Tepid Sponging:
Defined as sponging the skin with alcohol or cool water to lower body temperature during fever episodes.

The water temperature is maintained at 32°C (below body temperature) to facilitate rapid heat removal due to alcohol evaporation.
Sponge each area for 2-3 minutes, changing the washcloth, and monitor vital signs every 15 minutes.
Discontinue if the patient exhibits signs of discomfort or distress.

Temperature of Hot Water Bottle:
For normal adults: 52°C; for debilitated patients or children under 2 years: 40.5-46°C.

Local Application of Cold and Heat:

Application of Cold:
Can be administered in moist or dry forms, providing systemic and local effects.

Moist Cold:
Utilized in cold compresses, with a cloth immersed in cold water and applied to areas with large superficial vessels.

Dry Cold (Ice Bag):
Ice is placed in a bag, covered with a cloth, and applied to the affected area, maintaining a temperature below 15°C.

Application of Heat Purpose:
- Relieve stasis of blood and promote absorption of inflammatory products.
- Alleviate muscle stiffness and pain.
- Aid in the resolution of localized inflammation.
- Enhance blood circulation and promote suppuration.
- Provide warmth to the body.

Methods of Heat Application:

Dry Heat:
Using hot water bags, ensuring the temperature remains above 46°C for normal adults.

Moist Heat:
Administered via hot compresses, with a washcloth immersed in water at 40-46°C.

Complications:
May include paralysis, numbness, or loss of sensation due to fear of burns.

Sitz Bath:
Designed to soak the pelvic area, the patient sits in a tub or basin, immersing the area from the mid-thighs to the iliac crests or umbilicus.

Water temperature ranges from 40-43°C, unless the patient cannot tolerate it.

Purpose:

- Relieve pain in postoperative rectal conditions.
- Soothe irritated skin in the perineum.
- Aid in wound healing, particularly after episiotomy.
- Assist in bladder emptying for patients with urinary retention.

The duration of the bath typically ranges from 15-20 minutes, depending on the patient's condition.

Care must be taken to prevent burns, especially in elderly patients, when applying heat or cold therapy.

Study Questions:
1. Enumerate two purposes of heat application.
2. Describe the mechanism of action of heat therapy to achieve its objectives.
3. Define a tepid sponge bath.
4. Identify the common medication used in sitz baths.
5. Determine the average duration of time a patient spends in a sitz bath.

Body Mechanics and Mobility

Learning Objectives:

After completing this section, students will be capable to:

- Define the principle underlying proper body mechanics and its nursing implications.
- Enumerate the purposes of a range of motion exercises.
- Identify principles associated with safely moving clients in and out of bed.
- Demonstrate the safe transfer of a partially mobile client from bed to chair and vice versa.
- Demonstrate the teaching of various crutch walking gaits to a client.
- List different positions utilized for various examinations and treatments.

Key Terminology:
Body alignment, Dorsal lithotomy, Prone, Base of support, Foot drop, Protective device, Body

mechanics, Fowler's position, Recumbent, Center of gravity, Gait, Rotation, Contracture, Gait belt, Transfer belt, Centrolateral, Line of gravity, Sim's position, Dangling, Paralysis, Supination.

Acronyms:
AROM (Active Range of Motion), PROM (Passive Range of Motion), ROM (Range of Motion).

Body Mechanics: The strategic, coordinated, and safe utilization of the body to facilitate motion and balance during activities.

Proper Body Mechanics:
Utilizing the safest and most efficient techniques for moving and lifting objects, known as body mechanics, involves applying mechanical principles to human movement.

Basic Principles of Body Mechanics:

The laws of physics govern all movements, from which the following basic principles of body mechanics are derived:

- It is generally easier to pull, push, or roll an object than to lift it, with smooth and continuous movements preferred over jerky motions.
- Less energy is typically required to keep an object in motion than to start or stop it.
- Efforts should be made to work as close to the object as possible, utilizing strong leg and arm muscles while minimizing the use of weaker back muscles.
- Rocking backward or forward on the feet and using body weight can aid in pulling or pushing objects.

Principles underlying proper body mechanics revolve around three key factors: center of gravity, base of support, and line of gravity.

Center of Gravity:
Located in the pelvic area, approximately half of the body's weight is distributed above this point

and half below it, both horizontally and vertically. When lifting objects, bending at the knees and hips while keeping the back straight ensures the center of gravity remains over the feet, enhancing stability and balance.

Base of Support:
The feet serve as the base of support, with a wider base providing greater stability. Sideways stability is achieved by spreading the feet apart, while one foot slightly forward enhances back-to-front stability. Weight distribution should be even between both feet, with slightly flexed knees to absorb shocks.

Line of Gravity:
An imaginary vertical line passing through the top of the head, center of gravity, and base of support determines the direction of gravitational pull. For optimal efficiency, this line should be straight, ensuring equal weight distribution on each side and proper body alignment.

Body Alignment:

Maintaining proper body alignment during activities is crucial for balance and muscle coordination. Correct alignment ensures all muscles work together efficiently without strain. Proper posture, with weight slightly forward and supported on the outside of the feet, promotes alignment, akin to standing posture.

Positioning the Client:

Encouraging clients to move, whether in bed or walking, offers numerous benefits, including preventing complications associated with prolonged immobility and promoting self-care practices.

Moving and Positioning Clients:

These activities enhance comfort, restore bodily functions, prevent deformities, alleviate pressure, and stimulate respiration and circulation. Additionally, they increase muscle strength, mobility, and the patient's sense of independence.

Practice Guidelines:
- Maintain functional alignment.
- Ensure client safety.
- Reassure and comfort the client.
- Handle the client's body with care.
- Employ proper body mechanics.
- Seek assistance when moving heavy or immobile clients.
- Adhere to physician orders and avoid using special devices without authorization.

Turning the Patient to a Side-Lying Position:

Supplies and Equipment:
- Pillows
- Side rails
- Cotton blankets or towels (rolled for support)

Procedure Steps:

1. Wash hands and explain the procedure to the client.
2. Adjust the bed to a comfortable height and lower the client's head and side rail.
3. Move the client to the far side of the bed and raise the side rail.
4. Ask the client to reach for the side rail while assuming a broad stance.
5. Roll the client toward you, position their legs comfortably, and support their arms with pillows.
6. Wedge a pillow behind the client's back and adjust the bed height and head elevation.
7. Wash hands upon completion.

Joint Mobility and Range of Motion

Each joint in the body has a specific range of motion (ROM), which refers to its capacity for opening and closing movements. This range is delimited by points of resistance where further movement is impeded. Typically, individuals exhibit similar ROMs for major joints.

Passive Range of Motion

In cases where a client is unable to move independently, nurses administer passive range of motion (PROM) exercises.

Performing Passive ROM Exercises:

1. Wash hands.
2. Explain the procedure to the client.
3. Adjust the bed to a comfortable height and uncover the limb to be exercised.
4. Support all joints during exercise.
5. Execute slow, gentle movements during exercises, repeating each three times and halting if the client experiences discomfort.
6. Commence exercises with the client's neck and progress downward.
7. For the neck, flex, extend, and rotate it, supporting the head with hands.
8. For the shoulder and elbow, support the elbow with one hand and grasp the wrist with the other, performing movements such as raising the arm,

internal and external rotation, and flexion and extension of the elbow.

9. Perform exercises for the wrist and fingers, including flexion, extension, abduction, adduction, rotation, and thumb rotation.

10. For the hip and leg, support the leg while flexing, extending, abducting, adducting, and internally and externally rotating the hip and knee.

11. For the ankle and foot, dorsiflex, plantarflex, abduct, adduct, evert, and invert the foot.

12. Repeat exercises on the other side of the bed.

13. Position and cover the client, return the bed to a low position, and wash hands.

14. Document completion of PROM exercise.

Controlling Postural Hypotension:

To mitigate postural hypotension, sleep with the head of the bed elevated (8-12 inches) to lessen the severity of position changes upon rising. Avoid sudden changes in position and follow a gradual three-step process when arising from bed to stimulate renin production and prevent a drastic drop in blood pressure.

Balance is easier to maintain with minimal effort when enlarging the base of support in the direction of movement. Contracting muscles before moving an object reduces the energy required, while synchronizing the use of large muscle groups increases overall strength and prevents fatigue and injury.

The closer the line of gravity to the center of the base of support, the greater the stability, and greater friction against the surface beneath an object requires more force to move it. Moving an object along a level surface necessitates less energy than lifting it against gravity or up an inclined surface. Continuous muscle exertion can lead to muscle stretch and injury.

Body Positioning:

Positioning clients in various positions serves diagnostic and therapeutic purposes, promoting comfort, restoring body function, preventing deformities, relieving pressure, preventing muscle strain, restoring proper respiration and circulation, and facilitating nursing treatment.

Guidelines for Client Positioning

Ensuring Client Comfort:

Maintain optimal body alignment for the client, whether they are standing or lying in bed, to promote functional alignment and comfort.

Guidelines for Client Care

1. Ensure Client Safety: Prioritize the client's safety in all actions.
2. Enhance Comfort and Cooperation: Provide reassurance to make the client feel comfortable and willing to cooperate.
3. Handle with Care: Manage the client's body gently to avoid causing pain or harm.

4. Use Correct Body Mechanics: Apply proper body mechanics in all physical activities involving the client.
5. Seek Assistance When Needed: Get help when moving clients who are heavy or unable to move on their own.
6. Adhere to Specific Instructions: Follow all given instructions accurately.
7. Use Special Devices Only When Directed: Do not employ special equipment (such as splints or traction) without explicit orders.
8. Positioning for Examination and Treatment: Position the client correctly for any examinations or treatments.

Client Positioning for Examination and Treatment

Supine Position: Position the client lying flat on their back for examinations and treatments.

This position is commonly used for the majority of physical examinations. The client lies flat on their back with legs extended, and their arms are either folded on the chest or positioned alongside the body. A small pillow can be used for support. To maintain privacy, cover the client with a bath blanket. Note: Individuals with back issues may find this position uncomfortable.

This position is utilized for various examinations and procedures. The client lies on their back with knees bent and feet flat on the bed. Cover the client with a sheet or bath blanket folded once over the chest. Place a second sheet crosswise over the client's thighs and legs, wrapping the lower ends around the legs and feet. Fold the sheet to easily expose the genital area while keeping the client covered as much as possible.

Examining the spine and back is done in the Prone Position.
The client lies on their stomach with their head turned to the side for comfort. The arms can be positioned above the head or alongside the body. Ensure the client's privacy by covering them with a bath blanket. Note: This position is not

suitable for unconscious clients, pregnant women, individuals with abdominal incisions, or those with breathing difficulties.

Sims' Position: This posture is employed for rectal examinations. The client lies on their left side, typically with a small pillow under the head. The right knee is bent against the abdomen, while the left knee is slightly flexed. The left arm rests behind the body, and the right arm is positioned comfortably. Maintain the client's privacy by covering them with a bath blanket. Note: Clients with leg injuries or arthritis may be unable to assume this position.

Knee-Chest Position: This posture is employed for rectal and vaginal examinations, as well as for treatment to reposition the uterus. The client kneels with the chest resting on the bed and the elbows supported, or with the arms extended above the head. The client's head is turned to the side. Ensure that the thighs are perpendicular to the bed and the lower legs are flat. Caution: The client may experience dizziness or faintness and could fall. Do not leave the client unattended.

Crutch Walking

Crutches: Walking aids crafted from wood or metal shafts, extending from the ground to the client's armpits.

Application of Nursing Process
Assessment

Assessment:

Evaluate the client's physical capability to utilize crutches and assess the strength of their arm, back, and leg muscles.
Observe the client's ability to maintain balance.
Take note of any one-sided or unusual weakness or sensations of dizziness.
Determine which walking pattern is suitable for the client.
Assess the client's comprehension of crutch-walking techniques.

Planning/Objectives:

Enhance the client's ability to walk with lower extremity injuries.
Strengthen the muscles, particularly in the arms and legs.
Improve the client's sense of well-being through increased mobility.
Facilitate joint mobility.

Implementation/Procedure:

Educate the client on muscle-strengthening exercises.
Measure the client for properly fitted crutches.
Teach crutch-walking techniques: four-point gait, three-point gait, two-point gait, swing-to-gait, and swing-through gait.
Instruct on ascending and descending stairs with crutches.

Evaluation/Expected Outcomes:

Improved ambulation ability for the client.
Enhanced muscle strength in the client's arms and legs.
Enhanced sense of well-being for the client.

Teaching Techniques for Crutch Walking:

Four-Point Gait:

Equipment:
Properly sized crutches
Regular, solid-soled street shoes
Safety belt, if necessary

Procedure:
Explain the procedure's rationale to the client.
The gait is deliberate but offers excellent stability.
It's suitable when the client can bear weight on each leg.
Demonstrate the crutch and foot sequence to the client.
Move the right crutch.
Move the left foot.
Move the left crutch.
Move the right foot.
Assist the client in practicing the gait, offering support for balance as needed.

Monitor the client's progress and provide corrections as necessary.

P
Three-Point Gait

The equipment required is the same as for the four-point gait.

Explain the reasoning behind the procedure:

This gait is suitable when the client can bear minimal or no weight on one leg, or when the client has only one functional leg.
It involves a relatively swift pace and necessitates robust upper extremities and proficient balance.
Demonstrate the sequence of crutch and foot movements to the client.
Utilize two crutches to support the weaker extremities.
Distribute weight evenly on the crutches.

Advance both crutches and the affected leg forward simultaneously.
Follow with the unaffected leg.

Monitor the client's advancement and promptly address any errors.
Stay with the client until crutch safety is assured.

Demonstrate the crutch-foot sequence to the client:

This technique is a quicker version of the four-point gait.
It requires greater balance compared to the four-point gait.

Move the right foot and left crutch forward simultaneously.
Then, advance the left foot and the right crutch together.

Assist the client in practicing the gait and provide guidance as needed.

Evaluate the client's progress and address any errors promptly.

Teaching Swing-To-Gait and Swing-Through Gait:

Equipment needed:
Properly fitted crutches

Regular, hard-soled street shoes

Inform the client of the procedure's goal:

These gaits are typically utilized when the client's lower extremities are paralyzed, and braces may be used.

Demonstrate the crutch-foot sequences to the client:
- Swing-To Gait: Shift weight to the left and swing the body toward the crutches.
- Swing-Through Gait: Shift weight to the left and swing the body past the crutches.
- Bring crutches forward in line with the body and repeat the process.

Assist the client in practicing the gait and offer support as needed.

Evaluate the client's progress and provide corrections as necessary.

Teaching Stair Ambulation with Crutches:

Equipment required:
Properly fitted crutches
Regular, hard-soled street shoes
Safety belt (if necessary)

Explain the rationale behind the procedure to the client:

Ensure safety by applying a safety belt if the client is unsteady or requires support.

Demonstrate the procedure using a three-point gait:

Descending stairs:
- Begin with weight on the uninjured leg and crutches on the same level.
- Place crutches on the first step and transfer weight to the crutch handles while moving the unaffected leg to the step.
- Continue until the client is familiar with the process.

Ascending stairs:
- Start with the crutches and unaffected leg on the same level.
- Transfer weight to the crutch handles and lift the unaffected leg onto the first step.
- Shift weight to the unaffected leg and raise the other leg and crutches to the step.
- Repeat until the client understands the process.

Assist the client in practicing the technique, ensuring adequate balance, and be prepared to offer assistance if needed.

Evaluate the client's progress, address any mistakes, and document the following points:
- Time and distance of ambulation on crutches
- Balance
- Technique issues
- Remedial teaching requirements
- Client's feedback on the procedure

Helping the client into a Wheelchair or Chair:

Gather necessary supplies and equipment:

- Wheelchair
- Slippers or shoes with non-skid soles
- Robe
- Transfer aid (optional)

Procedure:

Explain the process to the patient and position the wheelchair appropriately next to the bed.

Prepare the client for movement, ensuring they are wearing a robe and slippers if needed.

Assist the client to sit on the edge of the bed, supporting their head and neck while moving their legs over the side.

Assist the client in standing, using proper body mechanics and a transfer belt if necessary.

Guide the client to the wheelchair, ensuring they use the armrests for support as they sit down.

Adjust the footrests and secure the client in the chair, providing any necessary reminders or assistance devices.

Cover the client with a blanket, provide access to the nurse call button, and wash your hands.

Monitor the client regularly and document the transfer process and their response.

Study Questions:

Identify the principle of proper body mechanics and its relevance to nursing care.
State the objectives of a range of motion exercises.
List principles related to the safe movement of clients in and out of bed.
Demonstrate the safe transfer of a partially mobile client from bed to chair and back.
Teach each crutch walking gait to a client.
Enumerate various positions used for different examinations and treatments.

Nutrition and Metabolism

Learning Objectives:

1. Describe the electrolyte composition of the body.

2. Define electrolyte.

3. Identify manifestations of fluid disturbance.

4. Describe causes of acid-base imbalance.

5. Perform procedures to maintain fluid electrolyte balance.

6. Apply procedures for ensuring nutritional maintenance.

7. Conduct proper NG tube insertion and feeding.

8. Assist in total parenteral hyperalimentation.

Fluid, Electrolyte, and Acid-Base Balance:

Fluid & Electrolyte Balance:

The body's normal function relies on a constant water volume and specific chemical compound concentrations (electrolytes).

Water – Vital for life, comprising 60-65% of body weight, essential for physiological functions.

Electrolyte – Compounds that dissociate in a solution, forming electrically charged particles (ions) – cations and anions.

Distribution of Body Water in Adults:

There are two main compartments of body water:

1. Intracellular fluid: about 40% of body weight (25 liters)

2. Extracellular fluid: about 20% of body weight (20 liters), comprising:

   - 5 liters intravascular

   - 15 liters interstitial (tissue space between blood and cells)

- Negligible amounts of other fluids like CSF, ocular fluid, synovial fluid, pleural fluid, pericardial fluid, and peritoneal fluid.

Water Balance:

Body water is dynamic, with constant loss and replacement, ensuring intake equals output.

Electrolyte Composition of Body Fluids:

Charged particles conduct electrical current in solutions. Example: NaCl dissociates into Na+ and Cl- ions.

Intracellular and extracellular fluids are separated by a semi-permeable cell membrane. Body fluids consist of water, electrolytes, and non-electrolytes, regulated by cellular actions.

Example: Na+ concentration is higher in extracellular fluid due to cellular actions known as sodium pump, which expels sodium from cells.

The major ions in cellular fluid, in order of quantity, are:

- Intracellular fluid (ICF): K+ (141 mEq/L), Mg++ (58 mEq/L), PO4++ (75 mEq/L)

- Extracellular fluid (ECF): Na+ (142 mEq/L), Cl- (103 mEq/L)

Transport Mechanisms of Electrolytes:

- Osmosis
- Diffusion
- Active transport (Na+ and K+ pump)
- Filtration
- Phagocytosis
- Pinocytosis

Osmolarity refers to the concentration of active particles per unit of solution, influencing fluid movement across vascular membranes.

Hydrostatic pressure of blood and osmotic pressure from blood proteins regulate fluid movement in and out of capillaries.

Osmotic pressure pulls fluid back into

capillaries, while negative hydrostatic pressure and interstitial osmotic pressure help suck fluid from plasma.

The result is the sum of outward capillary pressure and inward interstitial pressure.

Fluid Disturbances:

Fluid deficit (dehydration) occurs when fluid loss exceeds intake, caused by various factors like excessive sweating, vomiting, diarrhea, hemorrhage, or insufficient fluid intake.

Signs of fluid deficit include thirst, dry skin, decreased blood pressure, oliguria, acidosis, increased hemoglobin and hematocrit, weakness, apathy, and potentially coma and death.

Excess fluid can result from increased venous pressure, lymphatic obstruction, blood protein deficiency, capillary permeability increase, renal insufficiency, or excessive hormone production.

ACID-BASE BALANCE

Acids donate hydrogen ions, while bases accept them. The body maintains a pH balance of 7.35–7.45 through various mechanisms.

Acid-Base Regulation:

The body produces carbonic acid (H_2CO_3) from CO_2 and H_2O, regulated by carbonic anhydrase within cells. Cellular activity generates strong acids, requiring rapid neutralization or elimination.

Control Mechanisms:

- Acid-base buffer systems
- Respiratory regulation
- Kidney regulation

Buffers stabilize solution pH by converting strong acids or bases into weaker forms.

Respiratory regulation involves controlling carbon dioxide levels via lung exhalation.

Kidneys regulate acid-base balance by excreting $H+$ ions and forming bicarbonate.

Acidosis occurs when body hydrogen ion concentration increases and pH falls below

7.35, leading to respiratory or metabolic acidosis.

Respiratory acidosis results from hypoventilation, while metabolic acidosis may stem from diabetes, excessive alcohol consumption, renal failure, or dehydration.

Symptoms include restlessness, weakness, headache, confusion, and potentially coma.

Nursing interventions include improving ventilation, maintaining hydration, and monitoring vital signs and blood gasses.

Alkalosis involves decreased H+ concentration (<35 nmol/L) and pH above 7.45 due to carbonic acid deficit or excess bicarbonate.

Types include respiratory and metabolic alkalosis, with causes ranging from hyperventilation to medication side effects.

Symptoms include dizziness, muscle cramps, convulsions, and altered vital signs.

Nursing interventions include monitoring vital signs, encouraging slow breathing, administering CO_2 inhalations, and addressing underlying causes.

NUTRITION

Nutrition encompasses the study of nutrients and their utilization in the body, impacting overall well-being, behavior, and environment.

Nutrients are essential for growth, maintenance, and repair, with six classes: carbohydrates, fats, proteins, water, minerals, and vitamins.

The body cannot generate enough of these essential nutrients, thus food is the only way to consume them.

A healthy diet meets physiological needs and considers personal, social, and cultural factors, with no "good" or "bad" foods. Dietary Guidelines offer practical suggestions for healthy eating, aiming to meet nutritional needs, support activity, and reduce disease risk.

These guidelines are not individualized diets but serve as starting points for healthy eating plans.

To maintain a balanced diet, incorporate a

variety of foods into your meals as no single food provides all the essential nutrients needed. This variety also helps reduce the risk of nutrient toxicity and contamination. Ensure to balance your food intake with physical activity to manage or improve weight. Opt for diets rich in grains, vegetables, and fruits, while keeping fat, saturated fat, and cholesterol intake low. Similarly, moderate sugar and salt intake to reduce the risk of chronic diseases like hypertension, heart disease, and diabetes. Plant-based foods offer fiber, complex carbohydrates, vitamins, and minerals crucial for good health. Avoid high-fat diets as they increase the risk of obesity, heart diseases, and certain cancers. Foods high in added sugars contribute empty calories and promote tooth decay. Additionally, excess salt intake is associated with higher blood pressure levels.

Regarding therapeutic nutrition, it involves adjusting nutritional needs based on specific disease conditions or imbalances in nutrition status. This may include modifying diets to alter mineral, vitamin, protein, carbohydrate, fat, fluid, and texture components.

Gastrostomy and jejunostomy feedings entail delivering liquid nourishment through surgically inserted tubes, either into the stomach (gastrostomy) or the jejunum (jejunostomy). While typically temporary, they may become permanent in cases of esophageal obstruction.

For nasogastric tube insertion, ensure patient comfort and cooperation. Position them appropriately, select the nostril with better airflow, and prepare the tube accordingly. Mark its insertion length, lubricate it, and gently insert it into the selected nostril, directing it towards the throat. Advance it gradually, monitoring patient response and adjusting as necessary. Confirm correct placement by testing stomach contents acidity and auscultating air insufflation. Secure the tube and document relevant information for future care.

Nasogastric tube feeding requires determining feeding type, amount, and frequency beforehand. Administer feedings carefully, monitor residuals, and ensure proper tube care to prevent complications.

In order to avoid passing via the digestive system, parenteral nutrition entails injecting nutrients intravenously. It's crucial for individuals unable to ingest nutrients conventionally, but it requires specialized handling and is typically more expensive.

When assisting with catheter insertion, maintain sterility, ensure correct placement, and monitor for any complications. Evaluate the effectiveness of the procedure and ensure the patient receives necessary nutrients for tissue repair and sustenance.

Enemas serve various purposes such as cleansing, retention, and therapeutic interventions. Administer them with caution, considering factors like solution type, temperature, and patient's ability to retain the solution. Document the procedure accurately and monitor patient response closely for any adverse effects.

Flatulence Reduction Procedure and Urinary Catheterization Technique

Objective:

- To mitigate flatulence and reduce severe abdominal distention

- Preparation before administering a retention enema

Procedure:

1. The patient should be positioned on their left side.

2. Apply lubrication to the tube approximately 15 centimeters.

3. Insert the tube into the rectum, ensuring it penetrates 12-15 centimeters, and secure it with tape.

4. Connect the free end of the tube to additional tubing using a glass connector.

5. Ensure the end of the tube reaches the solution in the bowel.

6. Observe the amount of air passing by

noting bubbles in the solution. Optionally, attach a funnel to the free end of the tube and immerse it in an antiseptic solution in the bowel.

7. Educate the patient to avoid flatulence-inducing substances.

8. Leave the rectal tube in place for a maximum of 20 minutes to prevent prolonged effects on sphincter control.

9. Reinsert the rectal tube every 2-3 hours if distention persists or recurs, facilitating gas movement towards the rectum.

Urinary Catheterization:

Definition:

Catheterization involves introducing a tube (catheter) through the urethra into the urinary bladder and should only be performed when absolutely necessary to minimize infection and trauma risks.

Notes:

- Maintain strict sterility throughout the

procedure, following aseptic techniques.

Types of Catheters:
- Straight (plain or Robinson)
- Retention (Foleys, indwelling)

Selection Criteria:
- Choose catheter material based on estimated catheterization duration:
  - Plastic (up to 1 week)
  - Latex (2-3 days)
  - Silicone (2-3 months)
  - Polyvinyl chloride (PVC) (4-6 months)
- Select catheter size based on the diameter of the lumen, typically graded on the French scale or number.
- Catheter size depends on the urethral canal size:
  - # 8-10 Fr for children
  - # 14-16 Fr for adult females
  - # 18 Fr for adult males

Determine Appropriate Catheter Length:
- 40 cm catheter for adult males
- 22 cm catheter for adult females

Select Suitable Balloon Size:
- 5 ml for adults
- 3 ml for children

Straight Catheterization Purpose:
- Relieve bladder distention discomfort
- Assess residual urine
- Obtain urine specimen
- Empty bladder pre-surgery

Equipment Needed:
- Sterile catheter
- Kidney dish
- Galipot
- Gauze
- Towel
- Solution

- Lubricant

	•	Syringe
	•	Water
	•	Specimen bottle
	•	Gloves
II.	**Clean** •	Waste receiver
	•	Rubber sheet
	•	Flash light
	•	Measuring jug
	•	Screen

Preparing the Patient and Equipment for Perineal Wash:

Steps:

1. Position the patient in dorsal recumbent position, with the option to elevate the buttocks using pillows for females.

2. Drape the patient appropriately.

3. Clean the perineal area using warm water and soap, followed by rinsing and drying.

4. Set up the equipment and create a sterile field.

5. Drape the patient with a sterile drape.

6. Apply antiseptic solution to the area.

7. Lubricate the catheter insertion tip (5-7 cm).

Specific Techniques:

- For females, adequately expose the urinary meatus by retracting the tissue or labia minora upward.

- For uncircumcised males, retract the foreskin.

- Hold the penis firmly behind the glans and straighten it downward to facilitate catheter insertion, ensuring the catheter is held 5 cm from the insertion tip.

- Insert the catheter into the urethral orifice, 5 cm in females and 20 cm in males, or until urine is observed.

- Collect about 30 ml of urine for the specimen.

- Pinch any previous leakage.

- Drain the bladder and remove the catheter, following specific orders for adults with urinary retention.

Notes:

- If encountering resistance during insertion, avoid forcing it, as this can cause trauma. Encourage deep breaths from the patient to relax the external sphincter.

- Dorsal recumbent position offers better visibility of the urinary meatus in females and facilitates catheter insertion in males by relaxing abdominal and perineal muscles.

Retention (Indwelling) Catheter Insertion:

Purpose:
- Manage incontinence
- Provide intermittent or continuous bladder drainage and irrigation
- Prevent urine contact with incisions post-perineal surgery to prevent infection
- Monitor hourly urine output

Procedure:
- Explain the procedure to the patient.
- Prepare equipment: retention catheter, syringe, sterile water, tape, urine collection bag, and tubing.
- Inflate the catheter balloon to secure it within the bladder after insertion.
- Size the balloon according to the catheter size (5 ml – 30 ml).
- Insert the catheter slightly beyond the point of urine flow to ensure proper placement in the bladder.
- Inflate the balloon with a pre-filled syringe

and secure the catheter with tape.

- Ensure effective drainage and elevate the urine collection bag off the floor to prevent contamination.

- Document relevant data.

Removal:

- Withdraw the solution or air from the balloon using a syringe and remove the catheter gently.

Medication Administration

Learning Objectives

After completing this section, students will be capable to:

- Explain different methods of drug administration.

- Outline general guidelines and precautions for administering medications.

- Recognize the components and variations of syringes and needles.

- Identify essential equipment needed for medication administration.

- Discuss the importance of the five rights before administering drugs.

- Locate various sites for parenteral drug administration.

- Demonstrate the necessary steps for medication administration.

- Enumerate precautions to take during medication administration.

Key Terminology		
ampule	ophthalmic	parenteral
brand name	pharmacokinetics	trade name
capsule	pharmacology	transdermal
chemical name	potentiating	toxicity
dosage	prescription	transfusion
enteric coated	synergistic	vial
generic name	otic	z-track

Pharmacology delves into the study of drugs, which are chemical compounds capable of altering the functions of living organisms. Therapeutic agents, or medications, when introduced into an organism, modify its physiological functions.

Drug Metabolism:

The human body processes drugs through

four primary stages: absorption, transportation, biotransformation, and excretion. To achieve complete metabolism, a drug must be administered in a concentration adequate to produce the desired effect on body tissues, resulting in a change in these tissues.

Absorption Routes:

Drugs are absorbed through various routes including mucous membranes, gastrointestinal tract, respiratory tract, and skin. Mucous membranes offer rapid and efficient absorption due to their high vascularity. Oral drugs are absorbed in the gastrointestinal tract, influenced by stomach pH, food content, and disease conditions, with most absorption occurring in the small intestine.

Parenteral routes, including intradermal, subcutaneous, intramuscular, and intravenous, offer direct and rapid absorption. Other routes include inhalation, sublingual, buccal, and topical administration.

Transportation:

After absorption, drugs are transported to their action sites. Some drugs bind to plasma proteins while others circulate freely, with the latter being pharmacologically active. Lipid-soluble drugs are stored in fat and slowly released into the bloodstream post-administration.

Biotransformation:

The body converts drugs into less active forms through enzymes, mainly in the liver, but also in other organs like the lungs, kidneys, plasma, and intestinal mucosa.

Excretion:

Drugs are eliminated from the body through various routes, primarily the kidneys, which filter and excrete both the drug and its metabolites. Other routes include exhalation, feces, saliva, tears, and breast milk.

Factors Affecting Metabolism:

Personal attributes, physiological factors, genetic and immunological factors, as well as psychological, emotional, and environmental influences, impact drug metabolism and responses.

Source and Naming:

Drugs are sourced from natural sources like plants, animals, and minerals, or synthesized in laboratories. They are assigned chemical, generic, and trademark names for identification purposes.

Drug Administration:

The route of drug administration influences its action on the body. It depends on factors like the drug's nature, quantity, desired speed of effect, and the client's condition.

Safety Procedures:

Adherence to the Five Rights—right medication, client, time, route, and dosage—is crucial during drug administration to ensure patient safety.

Nursing Process Application:

Assessment, planning, implementation, and evaluation are integral to safe medication administration, including assessing routes, drug actions, side effects, and accurate dosage calculations.

Different Routes of Administration:

Various routes like oral, topical, parenteral (intradermal, subcutaneous, intramuscular, intravenous), rectal, vaginal, and inhalation offer diverse options for drug delivery.

Oral Administration:

Involves administering drugs by mouth, using different forms such as tablets, capsules, syrups, tinctures, suspensions, pills, and powders, with specific equipment and procedures for each type.

Suppository:

Rectally administered for laxative, local sedative, or therapeutic effects, requiring specific equipment and procedures for insertion and monitoring.

Parenteral Drug Administration:

Includes intradermal, subcutaneous, and intramuscular injections, each with distinct equipment, sites, and procedures for administration.

These procedures and guidelines ensure safe and effective medication administration, promoting patient well-being and treatment success.

Procedure:

1. Follow the ABC of the procedure.
2. Organize the tray and bring it to the patient's room.
3. Prepare the medication and draw it into the syringe.
4. Expel any air from the syringe.

5. Select the injection site, typically an intramuscular location.

6. Divide the buttock using the iliac crest as a guide, then clean the upper outer quadrant with an alcohol swab.

7. Stretch the skin and administer the medication.

8. Withdraw the piston (plunger) to check for blood return, indicating proper placement; if blood appears, change the needle and site.

9. Administer the medication slowly into the muscle.

10. Upon completion, withdraw the needle and gently massage the area with a swab to aid absorption.

11. Ensure the patient is comfortable.

12. Properly handle and store used equipment.

13. Document medication details and monitor the patient's response.

Note: Use a long needle for intramuscular injections and maintain strict aseptic technique throughout. Avoid inflamed, edematous, or abnormal areas for injections.

Giving oxygen through a nasal catheter involves various types of catheters, including a fine catheter, a spectacle frame with rubber tubing, or two soft rubber catheters connected by a Y-shaped connection to the oxygen apparatus.

Equipment needed includes an oxygen cylinder with regulating valve and pressure tubing, Wolf's bottle, glass connection, fine catheters, lubricant, plaster, safety pin, and a tray with saline or water.

The procedure is similar to administering oxygen via a mask. Connect the fine catheter to the pressure tubing and adjust the flow rate to 6-7 liters per minute. Lubricate the catheter with water and gently insert it into the pharynx, ensuring it reaches the uvula without forcing it against any obstruction.

It's essential to remove and replace oxygen catheters every 8 hours to prevent mucous membrane irritation. Oxygen administered through a catheter should be humidified to avoid drying out the mucous membranes. This method allows patients to move freely and receive about 50% oxygen concentration.

Oxygen tents are used to provide a high-oxygen environment for patients when other methods are not feasible. Equipment includes a transparent oxygen tent with its apparatus, ice (if refrigeration is unavailable), a hanger for the tent, and a room thermometer if necessary.

During the procedure, ensure electrical appliances are removed from the room, post no smoking signs, and set up the oxygen tent correctly. Adjust the oxygen flow to maintain a concentration of 40-60% for the initial period and then regulate it according to the doctor's orders. Regularly monitor the temperature and record the patient's condition and oxygen flow.

Precautions must be taken when using

oxygen due to its combustible nature. Smoking and sources of ignition should be kept at least 3 meters away from oxygen equipment. Avoid applying alcohol to the patient's skin and lubricating the catheter with Vaseline or oil. Handle oxygen cylinders with care, and always check for airway obstructions before administering oxygen to prevent suffocation.

In summary, administering oxygen through nasal catheters and oxygen tents requires careful attention to equipment, procedure, and safety precautions to ensure effective treatment and patient well-being.

Wound Care

Learning Objectives:

- Distinguish between various types of wounds.

- Explain the objectives of wound care.

- Enumerate essential equipment for wound management.

- Perform dressing procedures for both clean and septic wounds.

- Administer care for patients with draining wounds.

- Demonstrate proficiency in wound suturing and irrigation.

- Apply and remove clips appropriately.

Key Terminology:

abrasion   laceration   wound

debridement   pressure ulcer

decubitus ulcer   puncture

exudates   surgical incision

The skin serves as a protective barrier against external hazards. When the skin's integrity is compromised, it becomes vulnerable to microbial invasion, leading to potential infection. Any breach in the skin's surface constitutes a wound.

Wound Classification:

A wound encompasses any disruption in the skin's integrity, whether accidental or intentional. Examples include abrasions (surface skin removal), punctures (stab wounds), lacerations (with ragged edges), and surgical incisions (intentional wounds made under sterile conditions).

Wound Healing:

The process varies based on tissue damage extent and occurs through first, second, or third intention.

- First intention healing involves minimal tissue loss, such as surgical incisions, where edges seal rapidly with low scarring and infection rates.

- Second intention healing occurs with tissue loss, leading to granulation tissue formation and delayed epithelial cell growth.

- Third intention healing entails delayed wound closure, often seen after surgery, allowing for granulation before closure, with scarring being common.

Clean Wound Dressing:

Purpose:
- Maintain wound cleanliness.
- Prevent contamination and injury.
- Secure locally applied medications.
- Immobilize wound edges.
- Apply pressure.

Equipment:
- Pick-up forceps
- Sterile bowl or kidney dish
- Sterile cotton balls
- Sterile gallipot

- Sterile gauze
- Rubber sheet with cover
- Antiseptic solution
- Adhesive tape or bandages
- Scissors
- Ointments or other medications
- Receiver
- Spatula
- Benzene or ether

Technique:

Utilize aseptic technique throughout the procedure.

Procedure:

- Explain the process to the patient.
- Prepare and organize sterile and clean equipment.
- Adequately drape and place the patient in a comfortable position.
- Remove dressing layers sequentially, ensuring cleanliness.

- Clean the wound and surrounding skin meticulously.

- Apply medications as necessary and dress the wound securely.

- Document wound status and ensure patient comfort.

Septic Wound Dressing:

Purpose:
- Absorb wound exudates.
- Apply local medication.
- Prevent pain, swelling, and injury.

Equipment:
- Sterile gallipot
- Sterile kidney dish
- Sterile gauze
- Sterile forceps
- Sterile test tube or slide
- Sterile cotton-tipped applicators
- Sterile gloves (if applicable)

- Rubber sheet and cover
- Local medication
- Spatula
- Receiver with disinfectant
- Probe and director (if required)
- Scissors
- Benzene or ether
- Bandages or adhesive tape
- Bucket for soiled dressings

Procedure:

Follow a similar protocol as for clean wound dressing, ensuring meticulous wound cleansing and proper application of medication. Prioritize clean wounds over septic ones to minimize cross-infection risks.

Dressing with Drainage Tube:

Purpose:
- Prevent hematoma or fluid accumulation.

Equipment:
- Sterile kidney dish
- Sterile gallipot
- Sterile scissors
- Sterile forceps
- Sterile cotton balls
- Sterile gauze
- Antiseptic solution
- Sterile safety pins (if needed)
- Cotton wool or absorbent
- Receiver
- Rubber sheet and cover
- Adhesive tape or bandage
- Dressing scissors
- Ointment, paste, or paraffin gauze
- Spatulas (if needed)
- Sterile gloves (if available)

Procedure:
- Explain the procedure to the patient.
- Prepare and organize sterile equipment.

- Position the patient and protect the bedding.

- Remove old dressing and cleanse the wound meticulously.

- Handle the drainage tube with care and apply medication as needed.

- Secure the dressing firmly, ensuring patient comfort.

- Document wound status and dispose of soiled dressings properly.

Wound Irrigation:

Purpose:
- Cleanse and maintain wound drainage.

Equipment:
- Sterile gallipot or kidney dish
- Sterile cotton balls
- Sterile gauze
- Sterile forceps
- Sterile catheter

- Sterile syringe (20 cc)
- Receiver (2)
- Rubber sheet and cover
- Solutions (e.g., H_2O_2 or normal saline)
- Adhesive tape or bandage
- Bandage scissors
- Receiver for soiled dressings

Procedure:

- Explain the procedure to the patient and organize the necessary items.
- Position the patient and protect the bedding.
- Remove old dressing layers and prepare for irrigation.
- Cleanse the wound with antiseptic solution, ensuring thoroughness.
- Administer irrigation solution gently, ensuring proper drainage.
- Dress the wound securely and document its status.
- Ensure patient comfort and cleanliness.

Suturing:

Definition:

The application of stitches to body tissues using surgical needle and thread.

Purpose:
- Approximate wound edges for expedited healing.
- Minimize infection risk.
- Enhance wound closure aesthetics.

Equipment:
- Sterile needle holder
- Sterile round needle (2)
- Sterile cutting needle (2)
- Sterile silk
- Sterile catgut
- Sterile tissue forceps

- Sterile suture scissors
- Sterile cotton swabs
- Sterile cleaning solution
- Sterile dressing forceps
- Sterile receiver
- Sterile gauze
- Sterile plaster
- Dressing scissors
- Local anesthesia
- Sterile needle and syringes
- Sterile gloves
- Fenestrated towel

Procedure:

- Explain the procedure to the patient and prepare the area.

- Ensure hand hygiene and don sterile gloves.

- Anesthetize the wound edges if necessary.

- Approximate fascia layer edges with catgut sutures.

- Suture outer skin layer with silk, ensuring

proper alignment.

- Clean the wound, apply iodine, and dress it.

- Ensure patient comfort and cleanliness, and document wound status.

Stitch Removal:

Technique:
Employ aseptic technique throughout.

Principles:
- Remove sutures sequentially, avoiding fragmentation.

- Lift sutures for easier removal and ensure thorough cleansing.

- Dispose of removed sutures properly.

- Cleanse the wound surroundings and apply dressing as needed.

- Ensure patient comfort and cleanliness, and document the wound status.

Clips:

Definition:

Metal sutures used for skin closure.

Purpose:

Similar to suturing with stitches.

Equipment:

- Michel clip applier
- Clips
- Toothed dissecting forceps
- Cleaning materials (same as for suturing with stitches)

Procedure:

- Follow similar initial steps as for suturing with stitches.
- Instead of suturing, apply clips using the applier.
- During clip removal, maintain aseptic technique and ensure thorough cleansing.
- Document the wound status and ensure

patient comfort and cleanliness.

Study Questions:

- Identify various wound care methods.
- List three types of wound healing intentions.
- Enumerate purposes of septic wound dressing.
- Describe the suturing process.
- Define

Perioperative Nursing Care (Pre & Postoperative Nursing Care)

Learning Objectives:

- Enumerate preoperative preparation steps.

- Recognize high-risk surgical patients.

- Detail essential assessment skills for the preoperative, intraoperative, and postoperative phases.

- Clarify the significance of informed consent.

- Execute standard postoperative procedures including vital signs acquisition, consciousness level assessment, and surgical pain evaluation.

- Document and report postoperative complications.

- Evaluate patient airway status.

Preoperative Preparation:

Prepare patients for surgery by following specific steps tailored to their individual needs and the surgical procedure.

Identification of High-Risk Patients:

Identify patients who may be at increased risk during surgery due to underlying health conditions or other factors.

Assessment Skills:

Develop proficiency in assessing patients before, during, and after surgery, including vital signs monitoring, consciousness evaluation, and pain assessment.

Informed Consent:

Ensure patients fully understand the nature of the surgical procedure, its risks, benefits, and alternatives, and obtain their informed consent prior to surgery.

Postoperative Measures:

After surgery, conduct routine procedures such as monitoring vital signs, assessing consciousness levels, and managing surgical pain to ensure patient comfort and stability.

Documentation of Complications:

Document any postoperative complications accurately and promptly to facilitate appropriate intervention and follow-up care.

Airway Assessment:

Assess the patient's airway to ensure proper breathing and oxygenation before, during, and after surgery to prevent respiratory complications.

Key terminology		
anesthesia	hypothermia	postoperative
atelectasis	hypoxia	preoperative
elective	intraoperative	suture
embolus	perioperative	
evisceration	pneumonia	

Preoperative Care – Nursing Process Assessment

Assessment Priorities:

- Gathering nursing history
- Assessing the client's comprehension of the proposed surgical procedure
- Reviewing past surgical experiences
- Addressing fears, such as fear of the unknown, pain, death, or changes in body image
- Identifying factors contributing to surgical risk or postoperative complications
- Evaluating coping mechanisms and support systems
- Considering relevant socio-cultural factors
- Recording vital signs on the morning of surgery, noting any deviations
- Recording accurate height and weight, especially for pediatric patients
- Conducting a comprehensive review of systems
- Documenting results of all preoperative

diagnostic tests

Possible Nursing Diagnosis:
- Anxiety
- Ineffective coping
- Decisional conflict
- Fear
- Anticipated grieving
- Deficient knowledge
- Powerlessness

Planning/Objectives:
Before surgery, the client should:
- Demonstrate physical readiness for surgery, including normal vital signs and absence of infection signs
- Express any concerns or fears regarding the surgery
- Provide informed consent
- Demonstrate proper techniques for turning, deep breathing, and using equipment
- Understand the postoperative pain

management program

- Understand the postoperative activity plan

- Ensure the presence of adequate caregivers at home after discharge

Implementation:

- Establish a supportive nurse-client relationship

- Develop and implement a teaching plan to familiarize the client and family with the surgical process and pain management program

- Instruct the client on deep breathing, coughing exercises, and turning in bed

- Counsel the client and family on coping strategies and available resources

- Manage nutrition and hydration, ensuring compliance with fasting guidelines

- Assess bowel status and administer necessary bowel elimination interventions

- Perform preoperative skin and hygiene care

- Promote sleep and rest in the preoperative period

Evaluation:

Assess the adequacy of the care plan by evaluating the client's achievement of goals, including physical and mental readiness for surgery, understanding of postoperative care, and smooth recovery progress.

Pre-operative Purpose:

- Emotionally, mentally, and physically prepare the patient for surgery
- Prevent complications before, during, and after surgery

Equipment:

As necessary

Procedure:

- Ensure the patient's physical well-being before surgery through proper diet, hydration, sleep, and rest
- Address the patient's mental state by alleviating fears and explaining the surgical

procedure and safety measures

Day before surgery:

Physical preparation:

- Provide a complete bed bath, paying special attention to cleanliness and grooming

- If surgery involves the head, ensure thorough hair washing and shaving if necessary

- Administer ordered enema and document results

Psychological preparation:

- Briefly explain the surgery to the patient if they don't understand

- Ensure a good night's sleep for the patient, and report any sleep difficulties to the doctor

- Obtain informed consent for the surgery

- Instruct the patient on deep breathing and cough exercises

Day of Surgery:

- Ensure early preparation for morning

surgeries

- Enforce NPO status after midnight for morning surgeries; adjust food and fluid intake accordingly for afternoon surgeries

- Verify cleanliness and grooming, including shaving the operative area if needed

- Administer premedication as ordered

- Assist the patient onto the stretcher, ensuring safety and comfort

- Reassure the patient and ensure all necessary documentation accompanies them to the operating room

Shaving Purpose:

To reduce the risk of infection by minimizing bacterial presence on the skin

Equipment:
- Basin of warm water
- Washcloth
- Towel
- Soap
- Blade and razor holder

- Scissors

- Rubber sheet and towel

Procedure:

- Prepare equipment and position the patient comfortably

- Wash and shave the designated area, ensuring thorough cleaning and hair removal

- Follow specific instructions for different surgical sites to ensure cleanliness and safety

Intraoperative Nursing Care:

- Observation of surgical procedures to understand the process and support the patient emotionally

- Assist surgeons as either sterile or circulating nurses, performing tasks within or outside the sterile field, respectively

- Act as a patient advocate and maintain safety in the operating room

Post-operative Care Purpose:

- Prevent complications from anesthesia

- Detect signs of postoperative complications
- Support patient rehabilitation

Equipment:
As necessary

Procedure:
- Prepare the post-anesthesia care unit
- Assist with patient transfer and positioning
- Regularly check vital signs and evaluate the state of the patient
- Encourage coughing and deep breathing exercises
- Check dressing for bleeding or drainage
- Monitor tubing and drainage systems
- Provide comfort measures and pain management
- Limit visitors and follow postoperative orders carefully

Specific Post-operative Care:
Tailor care to specific surgical procedures,

addressing unique needs and precautions for each type of surgery

End-of-Life Care and Postmortem Care

Learning Objectives:

By the end of this section, learners will be able to:

- Identify the stages experienced by a dying person
- Define death
- Recognize signs of death
- Confirm death in collaboration with a physician
- Provide reassurance to relatives of the dying patient
- Administer respectful care for the deceased body
- Coordinate the transfer of the deceased body to the morgue or their home

Key Terminology:

Autopsy, Cheyne-Stokes respiration, postmortem examination, brain death, Kussmaul's breathing

Care of the Dying:

Death is a natural part of life, signifying the cessation of all vital processes. Legal death is defined as the complete absence of brain activity, as assessed and confirmed by a physician.

Spirituality and Death:

Death often prompts individuals to contemplate profound questions about life's meaning, the existence of the soul, and the possibility of an afterlife. Spirituality serves as a foundation for many facing death, providing strength, comfort, and support through various beliefs and practices, including drawing strength from God, prayer, and nurturing relationships with others.

Stages of Dying:

Elisabeth Kubler-Ross outlined five stages of dying, resembling the grieving process:

1. Denial

2. Anger

3. Bargaining

4. Depression

5. Acceptance

Nursing Process Assessment:

- Observe physical symptoms and signs of deterioration

- Assess the client's ability to meet basic needs independently

- Evaluate the nature and severity of pain

- Monitor for impending crises or emergencies

- Assess the client's psychosocial condition, including anxiety, sleep disturbances, and depression

Planning/Objectives:

- Assist the dying client in coping with the dying process

- Address personal feelings of loss and sadness while caring for dying clients

- Provide support to both the client and their

family throughout the dying process

- Complete necessary actions for caring for the deceased client

Implementation/Procedure:

- Minimize client discomfort
- Provide physical care, warmth, and assistance with hygiene
- Give prescription drugs for pain relief as needed.
- Recognize and respond to symptoms of urgency or emergency
- Support emotional needs through relationship-building, presence, and active listening
- Respect client privacy and autonomy, allowing for self-expression and solitude as desired

Care After Death:

Postmortem care involves respectful handling of the deceased body, including:

- Noting the time of death and notifying the

physician if necessary

- Performing hygiene tasks, such as closing eyes and cleaning the body

- Ensuring privacy and dignity for the deceased and their family

- Documenting all procedures performed

Study Questions:

- Define death and describe its stages
- Explain how death is confirmed
- Discuss the purposes of postmortem care

GLOSSARY

Abrasion: The act of scraping or rubbing off the skin.

Airborne precaution: Safety measures taken when a person has an illness that can be transmitted through the air or dust particles. This often involves special air handling and ventilation.

Ambulatory: Referring to the ability to walk.

Ampule: A small, sealed glass flask typically containing medication.

Anesthesia: The partial or complete loss of sensation.

Anuria: The complete suppression of urine secretion in the kidney.

Apex: The lower point of the heart, typically formed by the tip of the left ventricle.

Apical pulse: The pulse normally heard at the heart's apex, providing the most accurate assessment of pulse rate.

Aspiration: The inhalation of food, vomit, or saliva into the lungs.

Axilla: The armpit area.

Autoclave: Equipment used to decontaminate materials by exposing them to steam under pressure.

Apnea: The absence or lack of breathing.

Anoxia: A deficiency of oxygen in the tissues.

Asphyxia: A condition caused by prolonged lack of oxygen.

Asepsis: The complete absence of microorganisms.

Antiseptic: Chemical substances that can kill microorganisms or prevent their multiplication without causing harm.

Aplastic anemia: Anemia resulting from the destruction of bone marrow cells.

Atelectasis: A partial or complete collapse of the lung.

Aseptic technique: Procedures employed to prevent microorganisms from reaching surgical sites.

Auscultation: Listening to internal body sounds to identify abnormal conditions.

Autopsy: Examination of a body after death.

Base of support: The area providing stability or balance, typically the feet and their position.

Bed cradles: Frames placed over a patient's body or feet to support the weight of bedclothes.

Blood pressure: The force exerted by the heart to pump blood around the body.

Bradycardia: Abnormally slow heartbeat.

Bradypnea: Abnormally slow breathing, typically below 10 breaths per minute.

Brand name: The copyrighted name assigned by a company to a medication, also known as the trade name.

Brain death: The irreversible cessation of brain and brainstem function to the extent that cardiopulmonary function must be mechanically maintained.

Bounding pulse: A heartbeat stronger than normal.

Body mechanics: The use of safe and efficient methods for moving and lifting.

Carotid pulse: The pulse felt on either side of the neck, over the carotid artery.

Capsule: A small gelatinous case for holding medication or a membranous structure enclosing another body structure.

Catheter: A soft rubber tube used for the passage of fluids.

Center of gravity: The point where the weight of the body is evenly distributed.

Chemical name: The name of a medication that describes its chemical composition.

Cheyne-Stokes respiration: Breathing characterized by alternating deep breaths and very slow breaths or apnea, often preceding death.

Contaminated: An area containing germs or disease-producing material.

Constipation: Difficulty or infrequency in passing hardened bowel movements.

Contracture: Abnormal shortening of a muscle leading to deformity.

Cyanosis: Bluish discoloration of the lips, nose tip, and ear lobes due to lack of oxygen in the blood.

Cast: A material used to support and immobilize an injured part of the body.

Clips: Metallic materials used to hold skin together.

Closed bed: An unoccupied bed used when preparing a unit for a new client.

Congestion: Accumulation of blood or fluid in a part of the body, such as the lungs.

Contact precaution: Safety measures taken against diseases transmitted through direct contact.

Cystitis: Inflammation of the urinary bladder.

Dangling: Positioning a client so they sit on the edge of the bed with legs down and feet supported.

Debridement: The removal of foreign, dead, and contaminated material from a wound.

Decontamination: The removal of all traces of illness from an object.

Defecation: The act of excreting feces from the rectum.

Detergent: A substance dissolved in water used for cleaning.

Diagnosis: The determination of the nature of an illness based on clinical assessment and investigation results.

Diarrhea: Abnormal frequency and fluidity of bowel movements.

Diastole: The resting phase of the heart when it fills with blood.

Digitalis: A drug given to slow and strengthen the heartbeat.

Disinfectant: A chemical used to kill microorganisms.

Dorsal lithotomy: A position in which the client lies on their back with feet in stirrups.

Dosage: The amount of medication prescribed.

Dry heat: Air heated to high temperature for sterilization.

Droplet precaution: Safety measures taken to prevent the spread of diseases transmitted through droplets propelled through the air.

Dyspnea: Difficulty in breathing.

Dysuria: Painful or difficult urination.

Edema: Swelling due to fluid accumulation in body tissues.

Elective surgery: A non-life-threatening surgical procedure chosen by the patient.

Embolus: A foreign substance carried in the blood.

Enema: Injection of fluid into the colon or rectum.

Enteric: Relating to the small intestine.

Eupnea: Normal respiration.

Evisceration: The protrusion of internal organs through a wound.

Exhalation: Breathing out.

Exudate: Fluid that escapes from blood vessels and is deposited in tissue.

Fahrenheit: A temperature measurement system.

Femoral pulse: The sensation of a pulse above the femoral artery in the groin.

Fecal impaction: Accumulation of hardened stool in the rectum.

Fever: Elevated body temperature above 37°C.

Flatus: Gas in the intestines.

Footboard: A board at the foot of the bed to support the feet.

Foot Drop: A deformity preventing the client from placing the heel on the floor.

Fowler's position: A reclined sitting position.

Gait: Manner or style of walking.

Gastrostomy: Creation of an artificial

opening into the stomach for feeding.

Generic name: The name assigned to a drug by its first manufacturer.

Halitosis: Bad breath.

Hemoglobin: The oxygen-carrying pigment in blood.

Hypertension: High blood pressure.

Hypotension: Low blood pressure.

Hypothermia: Low body temperature.

Hypothermia blanket: A cooling blanket.

Hypoxia: Reduced oxygen in the tissues.

Incontinence: Loss of bladder or bowel control.

Infection: Invasion of the body by germs.

Inflammation: The body's reaction to infection or injury.

Infusion: Slow introduction of fluids into a vein.

Inhalation: Breathing in.

Intake: Fluid taken into the body.

Intraoperative: Occurring during surgery.

Irrigation: Injecting fluid into a

Dear Reader,

Thank you for reading Nurse's Toolbox: A Comprehensive Guide to Clinical Nursing Skills. We value your experience and would love to hear your thoughts. Please consider leaving a review on Amazon to share your feedback. Your insights will help us refine future editions and continue providing top-notch resources for the nursing community.

We look forward to your review!

www.ingramcontent.com/pod-product-compliance
Lightning Source LLC
Chambersburg PA
CBHW071458220526
45472CB00003B/849